PENGUIN BOOKS
Bathtime Bliss

Laura Jones is a fully qualified aromatherapist. She is kno..
for her innovative fragrant recipes and fresh contemporary approach
to aromatherapy and essential oils. She has studied traditional
aromatherapy and natural perfumery and works as a consultant
for leading aromatherapy and cosmetic companies.

LAURA JONES

Bathtime Bliss

PENGUIN BOOKS

Disclaimer

The use of essential oils by others is beyond the author's or publisher's control. No expressed or implied guarantee as to the effects of their use can be given, nor liability taken.

PENGUIN BOOKS

Published by the Penguin Group. Penguin Books Ltd, 27 Wrights Lane, London W8 5TZ, England. Penguin Putnam Inc., 375 Hudson Street, New York, New York 10014, USA. Penguin Books Australia Ltd, Ringwood, Victoria, Australia. Penguin Books Canada Ltd, 10 Alcorn Avenue, Toronto, Ontario, Canada M4V 3B2. Penguin Books (NZ) Ltd, Private Bag 102902, NSMC, Auckland, New Zealand · Penguin Books Ltd, Registered Offices: Harmondsworth, Middlesex, England · First published 2000 · Copyright © Laura Jones, 2000. All rights reserved · The moral right of the author has been asserted · Set in 10/13.5 Trade Gothic Condensed. Typeset by Rowland Phototypesetting Ltd, Bury St Edmunds, Suffolk. Printed in Great Britain by St Edmundsbury Press Ltd, Bury St Edmunds, Suffolk · Except in the United States of America, this book is sold subject to the condition that it shall not, by way of trade or otherwise, be lent, resold, hired out, or otherwise circulated without the publisher's prior consent in any form of binding or cover other than that in which it is published and without a similar condition including this condition being imposed on the subsequent purchaser · 10 9 8 7 6 5 4 3 2 1

Contents

Acknowledgements x

Introduction
xiii

What You'll Need   xiv

How Much to Use   xiv

Adding the Oils to the Water   xvi

Safety Check   xvi

Daily Living
1

Morning Recipes   4

Sunrise Special   4

Morning Glory   5

Jump-Start   6

Spring Essence   7

Crystal Clear   8

Instant Energy Dip   9

Double Courage   10

Decision Time   11

Evening Recipes 12
Revitalization 12
Out on the Town 13
Home Time 14
Sea of Relaxation 15
Camomile Calmer 16

Stress and Relaxation Stress Buster 20
17 Too Much to Do, Too Little Time 21
Liquid Calm 22
Emotional Soother 23
Spiritual Soother 24
Calm Before the Storm 25

Healing Baths Headaches 30
27 Stuffed Nose and Sinuses 31
Colds and Flu 32
PMT 33

Period Pains 34
Aches and Pains 35
Muscle Relaxer 36
Detox 37
The Morning After the Night Before 38
Winter Warmer 39
Summer Skin 40

Pamper Your Body Grace and Beauty 44
41 Pamper Me Softly 45
Slimmer's Soak 46
Body Toner 47

Purely for Pleasure River of Desire 52
49 Seduction Special 53
Passion Flower 54
Love You Tender 55
Absolutely Divine 56

Comfort Your Soul
57

The Angel's Bath   60
Vulnerable   61
To Mend a Broken Heart   62
Shock   63
Frustration   64
Fear   65
Confidence   66
Centring   67
Go with the Flow   68
Stillness   69
Creativity   70
Forest of Contemplation   71
Starlight Peace   72

Baths on a Budget:
The Five-Oil
Collection
73

Wake Up   77
Revitalizing   77
Relaxing   78
Bedtime   78

Aches and Pains   79
Breathing Free   79
Period Pains   80
Pampering   80
Seduction   81
Desire   81

Create your own recipes   82

Essential Oil Directory
85

Acknowledgements

I would like to thank everyone who people-tested the recipes included in *Bathtime Bliss* and those who gave me advice and feedback, especially Jenny Dufton, my editor, for her original suggestion and good-humoured help.

Essential oils can be found in some chemists, drugstores, pharmacies and health-food shops, as well as in specialist aromatherapy stores and on the internet; they can also be purchased by mail order. I have used the following companies' assistance with essential oils for the recipes in this book:

Earth Garden
2 Fairview Parade
Mawney Road
Romford
RM7 7HH

Telephone/Fax: 01708 722 633
Website: www.earthgarden.co.uk

and

Fragrant Pharmacy
Website: www.fragrantpharmacy.co.uk

Introduction

Lying back and relaxing in a bath is often one of the few opportunities we have to take time for ourselves. While you're bathing, why not boost the healing power of water by the addition of fabulous essential oils? These natural fragrant essences are the heart and soul of aromatherapy.

Pure essential oils are distilled from petals, leaves, fruits, seeds, barks, roots or wood — and one of the most beneficial ways to use them in aromatherapy is simply to add them to the bath. Science is now proving what fans of aromatherapy have long known – that the delicious fragrances can uplift your spirits, calm you down, prepare you for sleep, or rev you up for an exciting night out. The choice is yours! Essential oils can work on the mind, body and spirit – depending on the oil. Choosing which ones to use for particular moods or occasions is the key – which *Bathtime Bliss* provides.

How about a stimulating blend of essential oils to get you going in the morning, or a confidence-boosting blend if you're going for a job? You may want to choose oils to help rebalance your emotions if you're feeling out of sync, or to help you explore your spirituality. You may need a muscle-relaxing bath if you've just come in from the gym, but a different choice of oils will be called for if you want something sexy and seductive to kindle the fire of love. This is what *Bathtime Bliss* is all about — tailoring recipes to suit the occasion, and helping you enjoy life to the full.

What You'll Need

To become a fragrant water-baby, all you need is a few aromatherapy oils, a bathtub and water. Extra options are candles to set the mood, a favourite tipple – be it champagne or herb tea – your favourite music and, possibly, on romantic occasions, a special friend.

How Much to Use

You can use up to 8 drops of the *Bathtime Bliss* recipes in each bath, or as few as 4 drops – which will still have an effect. When you've found blends that work well for you, they can be pre-prepared. Put the essential oils in a small dropper bottle, using the same proportions as in the recipe, only in larger quantities. Instead of 2 drops, say, put 20. Instead of 3, put 30, and so on.

Although some people put essential oils straight in the bath water, others prefer to dilute them first in a small amount of vegetable oil, or even milk. I suggest you dilute the essential oils in a teaspoon of organic sunflower, grapeseed, hazelnut or almond oil. For those with dry skins, dilute the essential oils in 2 teaspoons of jojoba or avocado oil before adding to the water, and rub the floating oil into the skin while relaxing in the bath.

Adding the Oils to the Water

Run the bath about half-full, then pour your mixture in the running hot water, under the tap – just as you would a bubble bath.

Safety Check

* Certain essential oils are best avoided during pregnancy. Of those mentioned in this book, they include sweet basil, clary sage, ginger, Italian everlasting, juniper berry, marjoram, myrtle, nutmeg, rosemary and sweet thyme.
* People suffering from epilepsy should avoid using rosemary, which is often said to increase electrical activity in the brain (although to date no research is available to confirm this).

* Some essential oils can be irritating to sensitive skins if not well diluted. These include all the citrus oils, as well as sweet basil, cinnamon, clove, eucalyptus, ginger, hyssop, oregano, peppermint and sweet thyme. Anyone with sensitive skin, or an allergy to fragrances, should carry out a skin test twenty-four hours before using any new oil or recipe.
* Some vegetable oil or essential oils may affect acrylic or plastic baths if traces are left on the bottom or side of the tub.
* Essential oils should be stored in a dark, dry, cool place.

Daily Living

This section is divided into blends for the morning and blends for the evening because these are the times when most people take their baths. In the morning you usually want something to get you going, give you confidence, or in other ways help you get through the day; while in the evening you may want something to reinvigorate you after a tough day, help you to sleep, or put you in the mood for a hot date!

Morning Recipes

Sunrise Special

A Sunrise Special bath helps you greet the day with a calm, relaxed and positive attitude. You rise from it like a new dawn — smiling, undaunted, and ready to face whatever the busy day ahead may bring.

Bergamot	3 drops
Grapefruit	3 drops
Sandalwood	2 drops

Morning Glory

At work we need to feel confident in ourselves and focused. It helps if the brain is awake too. This blend of essential oils should help you sail through the day with ease.

Grapefruit	2 drops
Cajeput	1 drop
Lime	1 drop

Jump-Start

Ever had a day you couldn't quite get into, when you felt like staying in bed — preferably with the covers over your head? If you really do have to get up, this blend will give you the gentle jump-start you need. Slip into the bath and prepare to slide easily into another day.

Spearmint 2 drops
Rosemary 1 drop

Spring Essence

Imagine a bright spring morning, with the sun shining and the birds singing. You go to the windows and throw them open, full of the joys of life. This bath captures some of that spring vitality.

Petitgrain	2 drops
Ho-wood	1 drop
Palma Rosa	1 drop

Crystal Clear

Wouldn't it be great to be able to speak in meetings with total
clarity, get through the workload with impressive efficiency ... and
just a touch of inspiration? 'What's her secret?' they'll ask. Tell
them, but only if you want to give the advantage away!

Eucalyptus	1 drop
Lemon	1 drop
Rosemary	1 drop

Instant Energy Dip

Get energized with this revitalizing dip. Feel the buzz of
spearmint's verve, rosemary's vigour and grapefruit's vibrancy.
Nothing can stop you now.

    Spearmint   3 drops
    Grapefruit   2 drops
    Rosemary   2 drops

Double Courage

You need to be bold to get what you want out of life. Go out there with courage and a new daring that may even surprise you!

Lime	4 drops
Ginger	2 drops
Sweet Basil	1 drop

Decision Time

If you can't make decisions about anything, or feel as if you're somehow off-track and have lost the plot, this recipe should help focus your mind for the day ahead.

Tangerine	3 drops
Cardamom	1 drop
Geranium	1 drop

Evening Recipes

Revitalization

If you've just come in from a hectic day but need the energy to face an equally active evening, step into this revitalizing bath.

Lime	4 drops
Black Pepper	2 drops
Coriander	1 drop

Out on the Town

Put some pizzazz into the water – and get in the mood to party.
Perfect before a special celebration or exciting date.

  Rose Maroc   **4 drops**
  Tangerine   **3 drops**

Home Time

Feel like flopping out, lying on the sofa and taking it easy? No problem: this recipe will make it even more enjoyable.

Petitgrain	**4 drops**
Camomile Roman	**3 drops**

Sea of Relaxation

Linger in a sea of relaxation and let the worries melt away. Enjoy the warm embrace of the fragrant water and feel it ease the strain.

Clary Sage	2 drops
Orange	2 drops
Marjoram	1 drop

Camomile Calmer

Sleep like a baby and rise refreshed. Perfect for insomniacs and all grown-ups who need to be treated gently.

Camomile Roman	**4 drops**
Lavender	**2 drops**
Rosewood	**2 drops**

Stress and Relaxation

Stress saps your energy and holds you back, yet it's all too easy to become stressed-out. Life can sometimes feel like a hard slog with no respite — maybe because we have so many diverse areas to think about and deal with. If an additional strain is put on the situation, well, it can get very stressful indeed.

We all need to carve time out for ourselves so we can regain the strength we need at difficult times. Baths have always been a great way to do this, but add a few specially selected essential oils and you can practically feel the tension draining away.

Stress Buster

When you're feeling stressed, it's time to call in the stress buster!
The perfect relaxing bath to deal with everyday stress.

Orange	3 drops
Marjoram	2 drops
Lavender	1 drop

Too Much to Do, Too Little Time

This blend will help calm mental stress caused by nerves frazzled
because there's too much to do and not enough time to do it in.

Petitgrain	**4 drops**
Cardamom	**2 drops**
Palma Rosa	**2 drops**

Liquid Calm

Float in this pool of calm — and forget all your worries and
anxieties. Rebalance and re-energize, and stop fretting about
things that may never happen.

Camomile Maroc	3 drops
Lavender	2 drops
Patchouli	1 drop

Emotional Soother

When your emotions are fraught and your body is taut, breathe
deeply to take advantage of Mother Nature's soothing hand.

Rose	4 drops
Bergamot	2 drops
Geranium	2 drops

Spiritual Soother

Our spirit takes as many knocks as our body or mind, but the
essential oils in this blend will help you regain your spiritual
equilibrium.

Frankincense	4 drops
Camomile Roman	1 drop
Lavender	1 drop

Calm before the Storm

For those mornings when you just know it's going to be a stormy day ahead. This bath will help you feel calm and serene, prepared for anything

Orange	2 drops
Marjoram	2 drops
Clary Sage	1 drop

Healing Baths

The concept of healing baths has been explored since recorded history began, with health spas being enjoyed since Roman times. The recipes contain essential oils that may ease symptoms and reduce pain, and are known to have a beneficial effect on certain conditions.

Headaches

When your head is sore, dilute the recipe in half a teaspoon of vegetable oil, rub a small amount on the back of your neck and shoulders, add the rest to a bath, and relax the headache away.

Lavender	3 drops
Marjoram	2 drops
Spearmint	2 drops

Stuffed Nose and Sinuses

To clear the airways when your nose is stuffed up and you can't breathe freely, run the water, shut the bathroom door, and breathe in the healing vapours.

Cajeput	3 drops
Myrtle	2 drops
Rosemary	2 drops

Colds and Flu

To help take the edge off that horrible feeling when you think you might be getting the flu, take the bath, make yourself a nice hot warming drink, and snuggle up in bed. Things might look brighter in the morning.

Cajeput	2 drops
Frankincense	2 drops
Ginger	2 drops
Sweet Thyme	2 drops

PMT

You feel like shouting, the tension's mounting, and no one
understands. So run a bath, add the oils, and think of something
beautiful as the phyto-hormones in the geranium and clary sage
rebalance your hormonal chemistry.

Bergamot	2 drops
Clary Sage	2 drops
Geranium	2 drops
Tangerine	2 drops

Period Pains

Your belly feels bloated and sore, your back aches, and the only
thing you want to do is stay in bed. Try this — pour out half a
teaspoon of vegetable oil, add the essential oils below, and rub it
on your belly and back, then get in the bath. If that's too much
trouble, just add the oils to water and soak.

Geranium	**4 drops**
Italian Everlasting	**2 drops**
Lavender	**2 drops**

Aches and Pains

Your back is aching, you feel you can't stand up for another
minute, or get comfortable anywhere. You're getting tired and
irritable. What to do? Add the recipe below to half a teaspoon of
vegetable oil and rub it into any aching area before getting in a
warm bath. If you can't be bothered to do that, just add the oils to
the water and soak.

Rosemary	3 drops
Italian Everlasting	2 drops
Marjoram	2 drops
Cardamom	1 drop

Muscle Relaxer

The exercise class was tough, and now you regret pushing
yourself so hard. Add the recipe below to a teaspoon of vegetable
oil and rub it into your legs and arms before getting in a warm
bath. Alternatively, just add the oils to the water and soak.

Juniper Berry	3 drops
Rosemary	3 drops
Camomile Roman	2 drops

Detox

If your body feels sluggish and aches, if your brain feels heavy
and you've got no energy, it may be time to detox. Drink loads of
water to flush the toxins out, eat heaps of fruit and veg. Take this
detox bath every other day, over eight days, drinking a glass of
water both before and after the bath.

Cypress	2 drops
Juniper Berry	2 drops
Lemon	2 drops
Rosemary	2 drops

The Morning After the Night Before

If you're badly hung-over from a good night out, drink lots of
water, take a large dose of vitamin C and crawl into this bath.

Cajeput	2 drops
Grapefruit	2 drops
Juniper Berry	2 drops
Rosemary	2 drops

Winter Warmer

If you've just come in from the cold, soak in this Winter Warmer.
Afterwards, put your warm socks on, get your feet on the sofa, and
have a nice bowl of hot soup.

Nutmeg	3 drops
Ginger	2 drops
Myrtle	2 drops
Black Pepper	1 drop

Summer Skin

This blend can be added to a cool bath after a day in the hot sun.
The lavender cools, the camomile soothes the skin, and the
eucalyptus helps clear the head.

Lavender	6 drops
Camomile German	4 drops
Eucalyptus	2 drops

Pamper Your Body

Pampering is about being aware of your body and taking care of yourself in the most pleasurable way. No one needs a reason to use essential oil baths, just enjoy the experience of how good pampering can make you feel.

Grace and Beauty

Grace provides inner beauty, shining from within. It's a subtle thing that's got nothing to do with the shape of your nose. Grace is what pushes your shoulders back and holds your head up high. You float rather than walk — a goddess among women.

Petitgrain	2 drops
Rosewood	2 drops
Tangerine	2 drops
Ylang Ylang	2 drops

Pamper Me Softly

Be pampered by the sweet fragrances of this bath, gently lapping
against you, cosseting your body. To soften the skin, mix a
teaspoon of jojoba and avocado oil together, add in the essential
oil recipe, and gently massage the floating oil into the skin while
in the bath.

Ylang Ylang	3 drops
Geranium	2 drops
Orange	2 drops

Slimmer's Soak

Forget dieting. Just eat healthily, take regular exercise and your body will respond. This recipe is designed to help the body with the process of reduction. It helps reduce puffiness and that bloated feeling, while stimulating the body's metabolism into action.

Juniper	3 drops
Grapefruit	2 drops
Rosemary	2 drops
Coriander	1 drop

Body Toner

Toning, tuning, trimming ... if only shaping our body was as
simple as everyone tries to tell us. Until someone comes up with
an easy solution, eat a little less, exercise a little more, and use
this bath to help tone your skin. It's astringent, stimulating
and detoxifying.

Cypress	3 drops
Myrtle	3 drops
Grapefruit	2 drops

Purely for
Pleasure

When desire runs through a woman's body like a river drawn inexorably to the sea, men flock to her. It's like bees to honey — natural irresistibility. Unfortunately, we don't all have it all of the time, but nature has provided us with natural aphrodisiacs, many of which have been used by seductresses for centuries. Sexuality has many nuances. It can be tender or ardent, passionate or sweetly sublime, all aspects of the same eternal drive.

River of Desire

Awaken the river of desire within yourself. Feel it flowing ...
exciting, wild, uncontrollable. Laugh with the joy of it, and your
lover will yearn to join you.

Rose Maroc	6 drops
Lemon	2 drops
Nutmeg	2 drops

Seduction Special

Arouse and enrapture your lover with this Seduction Special. It's suggestive and inviting. You are sensual and soft. He is smitten. You are provocative and intriguing. He is besotted.

Rose Maroc	3 drops
Ylang Ylang	3 drops
Orange	1 drop

Passion Flower

Explore the inner landscape of your sexual self and find passion in unknown regions of your psyche.

Black Pepper	2 drops
Ginger	2 drops
Jasmine	2 drops
Rose Maroc	2 drops

Love You Tender

This bath makes you feel sweet and attractive, like a beautiful, delicate flower that can only be touched with the greatest tenderness and love.

Neroli	4 drops
Petitgrain	2 drops
Rose Bulgar	2 drops
Camomile Roman	1 drop

Absolutely Divine

Sometimes one oil is all you need to create a sexy bath and
sensuous atmosphere. The essential oils called 'absolutes' are
perfect for this effect – use rose, jasmine, tuberose or carnation.
Try adding 1 drop of black pepper to 4 drops of jasmine, or 1 drop
of patchouli to 4 drops of rose Maroc.

Comfort Your Soul

There are times in everyone's life when the comfort zone needed is so personal, it feels hard to express our needs to anyone else. These recipes help still the mind, rebalance the emotions, and awaken your spiritual self for creativity, intuition and enlightenment.

Angel's Bath

Immerse yourself in a celestial bath, to truly connect to the energy of your soul. Arise feeling blissful – a heavenly vision of inner beauty. Make way – an angel approaches ...

Jasmine	3 drops
Rose Bulgar	3 drops
Camomile Roman	1 drop

Vulnerable

When you're feeling fragile and vulnerable this recipe makes you
feel as if you're being held in big, strong, protective arms.

    Neroli   2 drops
    Rose Otto 2 drops

To Mend a Broken Heart

Nobody can describe the sorrow of a broken heart, which
pervades the mind and wrenches your soul. Find consolation
and inner strength in this bath. Time will heal.

Rose Bulgar	4 drops
Rosewood	2 drops
Lemon	1 drop

Shock

There are times when we feel shocked by life's events. It can be a positive jolt or a negative one, but either way the gentle fragrances of these flowers may help you deal better with whatever arises.

Geranium	5 drops
Lavender	3 drops
Rose	3 drops

Frustration

Frustration and anger can take you over, blinding you to what's really going on. That's why they say people can get into a 'blind rage'. Even if you feel there's something worth getting angry about, it's wise to have balance and be under control. This bath might help.

> **Clary Sage** 4 drops
> **Lavender** 2 drops

Fear

Most of us are fearful of something. It may be spiders. It may be
the bank manager. Sometimes it's nothing so specific, and what
you feel is really a lack of self-confidence and self-esteem. This
recipe should help calm your fears.

Jasmine	3 drops
Bergamot	2 drops
Camomile Roman	2 drops
Frankincense	1 drop

Confidence

There are times when we need our confidence to be shining
through — at a job interview, for example. Self-confidence inspires
others to have confidence in you.

Sandalwood	4 drops
Bergamot	2 drops
Geranium	1 drop
Palma Rosa	1 drop

Centring

Ever felt you were all over the place, kind of out of sync? You need centring.

Sandalwood	4 drops
Geranium	2 drops
Petitgrain	2 drops

Go with the Flow

Live in the present. Forget the past, stop worrying about the
future and enjoy the moment to the full.

Bergamot	2 drops
Camomile Roman	2 drops
Clary Sage	2 drops

Stillness

Still your mind, breathe deeply, and enjoy the silence that
stillness brings.

Cardamom	2 drops
Grapefruit	2 drops
Frankincense	1 drop

Creativity

Awaken your spiritual creativity, connecting into the universal
inspiration that is available to us all.

Petitgrain	4 drops
Grapefruit	1 drop
Ylang Ylang	1 drop

Forest of Contemplation

These aromas will transport you to the timeless temple of trees —
where you can contemplate life, and your part in it.

   Fir   4 drops
   Cypress   2 drops

Comfort Your Soul

Starlight Peace

Drift in the universal starlight. Close your eyes and be at one with
the dark blue immensity of peace.

Jasmine	2 drops
Rose Maroc	2 drops
Rosewood	1 drop

Baths on a Budget: The Five-Oil Collection

Because essential oils are so versatile, you don't have to possess a huge collection of expensive ones. A variety of different fragrant baths with diverse properties and uses can be created from just five oils. Just as in cooking, the secret is to choose the ingredients well, combine them in new and interesting proportions. A little more of this, a little less of that and – *voilà* – something new is made. And sometimes, a little goes a long way. Just one pinch of herbs can make all the difference to a dish, just as one drop of essential oil can transform a bath recipe.

For this collection, I've chosen five particularly useful and versatile essential oils. All are readily available wherever essential oils are sold.

* **Geranium** A soothing oil which eases anxiety. Also good for pain relief and to boost circulation. Used in skin care.
* **Grapefruit** This stimulating and uplifting oil blends well with many others. Please remember that as with all citrus essential oils, grapefruit may cause irritation in people with skin sensitivity. In such cases, a skin test is advisable.
* **Lavender** This is a good oil to use for stress relief and relaxation. As well as being very calming, and helping with sleeplessness, it's a natural antibiotic.
* **Rosemary** Another stimulating and uplifting oil, good for easing aches and pains and breathing difficulties. Please remember that it should not be used during pregnancy. People suffering from epilepsy should also avoid it.
* **Ylang ylang** Often used for seduction, this oil is very relaxing and soothing to the emotions. Used in skin care.

Wake Up

Grapefruit   5 drops
Rosemary   2 drops

Revitalizing

Rosemary   4 drops
Grapefruit   2 drops
Geranium   1 drop

Relaxing

Lavender	3 drops
Geranium	1 drop
Ylang Ylang	1 drop

Bedtime

Lavender	5 drops
Ylang Ylang	1 drop

Aches and Pains

Rosemary   5 drops
Lavender   3 drops

Breathing Free

Rosemary   6 drops
Grapefruit   2 drops

Period Pains

Geranium	6 drops
Rosemary	3 drops
Grapefruit	2 drops

Pampering

Geranium	3 drops
Grapefruit	2 drops
Lavender	3 drops
Ylang Ylang	2 drops

Seduction

Grapefruit	5 drops
Ylang Ylang	4 drops
Geranium	2 drops

Desire

Geranium	6 drops
Ylang Ylang	3 drops

Create Your Own Recipes

If you wish to achieve a particular effect, look through the Essential Oil Directory for an essential oil, or oils, with the relevant properties, and create your own recipe. By varying the amount of drops you use, you can combine these five oils in hundreds of different ways, which would be impossible to list. So do experiment — by changing the number of drops you use, or by putting together new oil combinations.

There is only one rule to remember: the

stronger the smell, the more it will overpower the gentler-smelling oils in your recipe. And one extra drop of an oil can change not only the fragrance of a recipe, but its therapeutic properties.

All these essential oils can be used on their own in a bath.

Essential Oil
Directory

(Sweet) Basil Linalol – *Ocimum basilicum*
Good for stimulating the mind, relaxing the body and easing cramps, pains and coughs while generally giving a feeling of well-being. (There are two types of basil – use sweet basil only as the other type may cause irritation when used in the bath.)

Bergamot FCF – *Citrus bergamia*
A wonderfully uplifting oil, good to use on days when you're feeling low. Known as an effective antidepressant. It's also a good antiseptic, and used in healing.

Black Pepper – *Piper nigrum*
Stimulating and warming, good for circulation, respiratory problems, colds, flu and aching muscles.

Cajeput – *Melaleuca cajeputi*
An antiseptic healing oil, good for coughs and colds, breathing difficulties and aching muscles.

Camomile German – *Matricaria recutica*
A dark bluish oil that can be used when the skin needs calming and cooling.

Camomile Maroc – *Ormenis multicaulis*
This is not a 'true' camomile oil, but it is soothing, antiseptic and healing. Good for relaxation, and to ease anxiety and stress.

Camomile Roman – *Anthemis nobilis*
A soothing, gentle, healing oil. Good for calm and peace of mind, to ease aches, pains and inflammations, and for skin care.

Cardamom – *Elettaria cardamomum*
Good for fatigue, digestion, stomach cramps, circulation, nervousness and feelings of coldness.

Clary Sage – *Salvia sclarea*
A really calming oil, good for nerves, stress, pain and anxiety.

Coriander – *Coriandrum sativum*
Good for exhaustion, stress and tension, and for general well-being. Use when a little uplifting is needed.

Cypress – *Cupressus sempervirens*
A healing oil, used for detoxifying and purifying. It's astringent, and good for varicose veins and fluid retention.

Eucalyptus – *Eucalyptus radiata & E. globulas*
A cooling oil that can be used to stimulate and awaken the mind. A good oil to use when the nose feels stuffy, and the air needs clearing.

Fir – *Abies alba*
Good to refresh and awaken, for coughs and colds, and when the body is aching. Most often used in room methods such as diffusers.

Frankincense – *Boswellia carterii*
Good for respiratory problems, coughs, colds and skin care. Uplifting and purifying, it also eases stress and tension.

Geranium – *Pelargonium graveolens*
A wonderfully sweet flowery oil. Uplifting and relaxing, it is also good for nervous tension, circulation, period pains, PMT and skin care.

Ginger – *Zingiber officinale*
Warming and stimulating. It is also good for exhaustion, colds and flu, helps boost circulation, and eases aches and pains.

Grapefruit – *Citrus paradisi*
Uplifting and stimulating. Use when you're feeling low and in need of perking up. Good for stress and tension, toning the body, and to promote well-being.

Ho-wood – *Cinnamomum camphora*
A soothing yet stimulating oil that is grounding. Use when the mind and body need to rest but not sleep. Good for skin care and healing.

Italian Everlasting – *Helichrysum angustifolia*
Helps ease pain caused by a bump or bruising, a period or muscle stiffness.

Jasmine – *Jasminum officinale*
One of nature's ultimate sexy, pampering fragrances. Used for skin care as well as for sensuality, it's good for relaxation and well-being.

Juniper Berry – *Juniperus communis*
Good for fluid retention, aches and pains, detoxification, cellulite and generally getting in shape.

Lavender – *Lavendula angustifolia*
The first oil to buy. Does just about everything. It's an antiseptic,
so can be used around minor cuts and grazes. It helps you sleep
and reduces tension and stress.

Lemon – *Citrus limon*
A very useful oil. Refreshing, uplifting and calming, it is also an
antiseptic and good for toning the body and skin care. Can be
blended with all essential oils.

Lime – *Citrus aurantifolia*
Generally uplifting and stimulating. Gives a sense of well-being.
Good in blends.

Marjoram – *Origanum majorana*
For relaxation, reducing stress and tension, and easing aches and pains. For those who are feeling anxious and unsettled.

Myrtle – *Myrtus communis*
A good healing oil, used for the relief of coughs, colds and tiredness. Also helps clear feelings of stuffiness.

Neroli – *Citrus aurantium*
This uplifting and relaxing oil helps dispel nervousness and anxiety. Often used in meditation and for contacting the inner self. Excellent for skin care.

Nutmeg – *Myristica fragrans*
Warming, comforting and soothing. Helps to reduce tension and
anxiety, and aches and pains.

(Sweet) Orange – *Citrus sinensis*
An uplifting, cheerful oil that brings a sense of well-being.

Palma Rosa – *Cymbopogon martinii*
Good for nervousness, anxiety and skin conditions that require an
antiseptic in the water.

Patchouli – *Pogostemon cablin*
This well-known antidepressant is used extensively in Asia as a cure-all and aphrodisiac.

Petitgrain – *Citrus aurantium*
This uplifting oil gives a sense of well-being and is particularly good for easing the stress of overwork. Helps when you're feeling exhausted.

Rose Bulgar or Rose Otto – *Rosa damascena*
A gentle fragrance that is comforting and soothing. Good for skin care, as well as love.

Rose Maroc – *Rosa centifoli*
This is the rose of seduction – heady, sexy and full of promise.

Rosemary – *Rosmarinus officinalis*
An awakening fragrance, very uplifting. Good for detoxifying,
cellulite and toning the body. Useful for general respiratory
problems, and aches and pains.

Rosewood – *Aniba rosaeodora*
Eases nervous tension, giving a sense of relaxation and calm
while being stimulating and centring.

Sandalwood – *Santalum album*
Use as an aphrodisiac as well as a healing oil. Good for nervous tension, stress, anxiety, skin care and toning the body.

Spearmint – *Mentha spicata*
Used for tiredness, and when a little stimulation is needed. Helps reduce headaches and eases overloaded minds and digestive problems.

Tangerine – *Citrus reticulata*
A relaxing and soothing citrus oil. Can be used for insomnia and stress. Also helps reduce fluid retention.

(Sweet) Thyme Linalol — *Thymus vulgaris linalol*
This is a very strong oil said to have antiviral properties, and to be able to help get rid of bacteria. Good for healing when something strong is needed. Often best used in burners.

Ylang Ylang — *Cananga odorata*
The exotic fragrance of this oil stimulates the senses. It's an aphrodisiac with calming and relaxing properties. Too much can be sedative.